# Somatic Exercises for Beginners

## Basic Somatic Exercises

By

Kincade Lonan

# Table of Contents

# CHAPTER 1

# Introduction to Somatic Exercises

## 1.1 What Are Somatic Exercises?

Somatic exercises are a unique approach to movement and body awareness that can transform the way we experience and inhabit our own bodies. At their core, somatic exercises are a means of enhancing the mind-body connection and promoting greater bodily awareness. Unlike traditional exercises that often focus solely on physical conditioning, somatic exercises delve into the subtleties of how we move, perceive, and experience our bodies.

Somatic exercises draw their name from the word "soma," which in ancient Greek refers to the living body as a unified whole. This concept is central to somatic practices. Somatic exercises are not just about building muscle or increasing flexibility; they are about re-educating the nervous system to release chronic muscular tension and regain optimal movement patterns.

These exercises are rooted in the work of Thomas Hanna, who developed a somatic education system known as "Hanna Somatic Education" in the mid-20th century. Hanna's insights into sensory motor amnesia (SMA) laid the foundation for somatic exercises. SMA is a condition in which the brain loses control over certain muscles due to habitual patterns of tension and stress. Somatic exercises aim to address SMA by facilitating the voluntary release of these habituated muscular contractions.

# 1.2 Benefits of Somatic Exercises

The benefits of incorporating somatic exercises into your daily routine are multifaceted and extend beyond just physical well-being. Here are some key advantages:

**1. Improved Body Awareness:** Somatic exercises cultivate a heightened sense of body awareness. By paying close attention to the subtle sensations in your body during somatic movements, you become more attuned to how your body functions and responds to various stimuli.

**2. Pain Relief:** Somatic exercises are renowned for their efficacy in alleviating chronic pain, particularly back pain, neck pain, and joint pain. These exercises address the root cause of many painful conditions—chronic muscle tension—and can lead to significant and lasting relief.

**3. Enhanced Flexibility and Range of Motion:** Somatic exercises promote flexibility and improved range of motion without the forceful stretching often associated with traditional exercises. Instead of forcing your body into a position, somatics encourage your muscles to release tension, allowing for natural and sustainable flexibility gains.

**4. Stress Reduction:** Somatic exercises emphasize relaxation and stress reduction. As you become proficient in releasing muscular tension, you'll notice a reduction in stress and anxiety levels. The mind-body connection fostered by somatic practice can lead to a calmer and more centered state of being.

**5. Improved Posture:** Poor posture is a common issue in today's sedentary society. Somatic exercises help address posture problems by resetting the neuromuscular patterns that contribute to slouching, rounded shoulders, and other postural issues. Better posture not only looks more appealing but also supports overall spinal health.

**6. Mind-Body Integration:** Somatic exercises encourage a harmonious connection between your mind and body. This integration can have a profound impact on your overall sense of well-being, emotional stability, and self-awareness.

**7. Sustainable Self-Care:** Somatic exercises empower individuals to take control of their own health and well-being. Once you learn these techniques, you have a valuable tool for self-care that you can use throughout your life to address physical discomfort and maintain optimal movement patterns.

somatic exercises offer a holistic approach to physical and mental well-being. By re-educating your body and mind to work together in harmony, you can experience significant improvements in your quality of life, from pain relief to enhanced body awareness and emotional balance. As we delve deeper into this topic in the subsequent chapters, you'll gain a deeper understanding of how somatic exercises work and how to incorporate them into your daily routine for maximum benefit.

# CHAPTER 2

# Understanding Somatics

## 2.1 The Somatic System

The somatic system is a fundamental aspect of human physiology, encompassing the body's sensory and motor functions, perception, and movement. It is essentially the bridge between the physical body and the mind, allowing us to sense, move, and interact with our environment. The term "somatic" is derived from the Greek word "soma," which means "body." In the context of somatic exercises and education, understanding the somatic system is crucial.

The somatic system includes various components:

- **Sensory Receptors:** These are specialized nerve endings distributed throughout the body, providing information about touch, temperature, pressure, proprioception (awareness of body position), and nociception (perception of pain).

- **Motor Neurons:** Motor neurons transmit signals from the brain to the muscles, enabling voluntary movement. The coordination of these neurons is essential for fluid and controlled motion.

- **The Brain and Central Nervous System:** The brain plays a central role in processing sensory information, making decisions, and sending commands to muscles. The central nervous system coordinates the body's responses to external stimuli and internal conditions.

- **Sensory-Motor Feedback Loop:** The somatic system operates as a continuous feedback loop, with sensory information informing motor actions and motor actions generating sensory feedback. This loop allows for real-time adjustments in movement and posture.

Understanding the somatic system's intricacies is essential for grasping the principles behind somatic exercises and how they facilitate improved movement and well-being.

## 2.2 Sensory Motor Amnesia (SMA)

Sensory Motor Amnesia (SMA) is a central concept in somatic education. It refers to the condition in which the brain loses awareness and control over certain muscles due to chronic patterns of tension and stress. This phenomenon often results from habitual responses to physical or emotional stressors, injury, or even long hours spent in fixed positions (e.g., sitting at a desk for extended periods).

SMA can lead to various issues, including chronic pain, limited range of motion, and compromised posture. Somatic exercises are designed to address SMA by reintroducing the brain to these forgotten muscles and restoring voluntary control. Through a combination of gentle movements, focused attention, and sensory feedback, individuals can learn to release the chronic muscular tension associated with SMA and regain optimal function.

## 2.3 The Mind-Body Connection

The mind-body connection is a fundamental principle underlying somatic exercises. It acknowledges that the mind and body are inseparable and that mental and emotional states can profoundly impact physical well-being. Conversely, the state of the body can influence mental and emotional states.

Somatic exercises emphasize the importance of cultivating mindful awareness of one's body. By practicing somatic with a heightened sense of presence and attention, individuals can break free from habitual movement patterns, reduce stress, and promote relaxation. The mind-body connection in somatic exercises means that improving physical function can lead to mental and emotional improvements, and vice versa.

## 2.4 Principles of Somatic Education

Somatic education is guided by several key principles, including:

- **Self-Responsibility:** Somatic education places the onus of learning and healing on the individual. It empowers individuals to take an active role in their own well-being, emphasizing self-awareness and self-regulation.

- **Slow and Gentle Movements:** Somatic exercises are typically slow and gentle. This approach allows individuals to tune into their bodies, feel for areas of tension, and release that tension gradually.

- **Pandiculation:** Pandiculation is a core somatic concept involving the intentional contraction and release of muscles. It serves as a fundamental technique for resetting muscle length and function.

- **Awareness and Sensation:** Heightened awareness of bodily sensations is integral to somatic exercises. Practitioners are encouraged to explore and feel subtle changes in muscle tension and movement patterns.

- **Mindful Attention:** Somatic exercises are performed with mindful attention, which means being fully present in the moment and focused on the sensations and movements of the body.

# CHAPTER 3

# Getting Started

## 3.1 Creating a Safe Space

Before diving into somatic exercises, it's essential to create a safe and conducive environment for your practice. Creating a safe space is not just about physical safety; it also encompasses mental and emotional comfort. Here's how to do it:

**Physical Safety:**

- **Clear the Area:** Ensure that the space where you'll be practicing is free from obstacles and hazards that could cause accidents or interruptions.

- **Appropriate Attire:** Wear comfortable clothing that allows for unrestricted movement. Remove any restrictive accessories or jewelry that might interfere with your practice.

- **Non-Slip Surface:** If possible, practice on a non-slip surface, like a yoga mat or carpet, to prevent slips or falls during movements.

**Mental and Emotional Comfort:**

- **Privacy:** Find a quiet, private space where you won't be easily distracted or interrupted. Turn off your phone or put it on silent mode to minimize distractions.

- **Time and Commitment:** Dedicate a specific time for

your somatic practice, and commit to it. Knowing that you have this time set aside can help reduce mental stress and allow you to focus fully on the practice.

- **Mindset:** Approach your somatic practice with an open and curious mindset. Release any judgment or expectations about your performance. Remember that somatic exercises are about exploration and self-discovery, not achieving perfection.

- **Support:** If you're new to somatic exercises, consider seeking support or guidance from a qualified somatic practitioner or instructor. They can provide valuable feedback and ensure you're practicing safely and effectively.

Creating a safe space sets the stage for a positive and productive somatic practice. It allows you to let go of external distractions and concerns, enabling you to fully engage with your body and the exercises.

# 3.2 Warm-Up and Preparations

Just like any physical activity, somatic exercises benefit from a proper warm-up. However, somatic warm-ups are distinct from traditional stretching or cardio warm-ups. They serve to prepare your body and mind for the somatic experience ahead. Here's how to effectively warm up:

**Mindful Breathing:** Begin with mindful breathing exercises to center yourself and shift your focus inward. Deep, diaphragmatic breaths help relax the nervous system and set the stage for mindful movement.

**Body Scan:** Conduct a gentle body scan. Start from your head and work your way down to your toes, paying attention to any areas of tension or discomfort. This preliminary body scan helps you become aware of your current physical state.

**Joint Mobilization:** Perform gentle joint mobilization exercises. These may include rotating your wrists, ankles, shoulders, and hips. These movements increase joint lubrication and prepare your joints for somatic exercises.

**Pandiculation:** Engage in pandiculation for specific muscle groups that will be the focus of your somatic exercises. Pandiculation involves contracting and then slowly releasing muscles to reset their length and function.

**Sensory Awareness:** Take a moment to focus on your sensory perception. Notice the sensation of your clothing against your skin, the temperature of the room, and any sounds or smells in your environment. This sensory awareness helps ground you in the present moment.

# 3.3 Breathing Techniques

Breathing is a fundamental aspect of somatic exercises, as it serves as a bridge between the mind and body. The way you breathe can profoundly influence your physical and mental states. Here are some essential breathing techniques to incorporate into your somatic practice:

**Diaphragmatic Breathing:**
Diaphragmatic breathing, also known as abdominal or belly breathing, involves using the diaphragm—a large muscle located beneath the lungs—rather than shallow chest breathing. To practice diaphragmatic breathing:

- Find a comfortable seated or lying position.

- Place one hand on your chest and the other on your abdomen.

- Inhale deeply through your nose, allowing your abdomen

to expand as you fill your lungs
with air.

- Exhale slowly through your
  mouth, feeling your abdomen
  contract.

- Focus on the rise and fall of
  your abdomen, keeping your
  chest relatively still.

**Three-Part Breath:** This technique
divides the breath into three parts: the
lower, middle, and upper lungs. It
promotes fuller, more balanced
breathing. To practice the three-part
breath:

- Begin with diaphragmatic
  breathing, filling the lower part
  of your lungs.

- Continue to inhale, expanding
  your ribcage to fill the middle
  part of your lungs.

- Finally, fill the upper part of your lungs by lifting your collarbones slightly.

- Exhale in the reverse order, starting with the upper lungs and gradually releasing the lower.

**Equal-Length Breathing:** Equal-length breathing involves making the inhalation and exhalation of equal duration, promoting a balanced breath cycle. You can use a simple count to achieve this:

- Inhale for a count of, say, four.

- Exhale for the same count of four.

- As you become more comfortable, you can extend the count to six or eight for a deeper and more calming breath.

**Mindful Breath Awareness:** This technique involves bringing your full attention to your breath. As you breathe, observe the sensation of the breath entering and leaving your body. Notice the rise and fall of your abdomen or the gentle movement of air at your nostrils. Whenever your mind wanders, gently bring your focus back to your breath.

Breathing techniques serve several purposes in somatic exercises. They help to:

- **Relax the Nervous System:** Deep, diaphragmatic breathing activates the parasympathetic nervous system, which promotes relaxation and reduces stress.

- **Enhance Body Awareness:** Focusing on your breath can help you tune into your body's subtle sensations and changes during somatic movements.

- **Facilitate Mind-Body Connection:** Conscious breathing establishes a direct link between your mental state and your physical experience, reinforcing the mind-body connection central to somatic exercises.

## 3.4 Mindful Awareness

Mindful awareness is a core principle of somatic exercises, emphasizing the importance of being fully present in the moment. It involves directing your attention to the sensations, movements, and experiences occurring in your body as you engage in somatic exercises. Here's how to cultivate mindful awareness in your practice:

**Focused Attention:** Concentrate your attention on the specific area or muscle group you are working on during each somatic exercise. Avoid distractions and maintain a singular focus on the sensations and changes happening within your body.

**Non-Judgmental Observation:** Approach your practice with an attitude of non-judgmental observation. Release any self-criticism or evaluation of your performance. Instead, simply notice what is happening without labeling it as "good" or "bad."

**Sensory Exploration:** Explore the sensations in your body as you move through somatic exercises. Notice areas of tension, warmth, tingling, or relaxation. Be curious and open to whatever you discover.

**Breath Awareness:** As mentioned in the previous section, pay attention to your breath. It serves as an anchor for your awareness, grounding you in the present moment and connecting you to the physical sensations of your body.

**Patience and Acceptance:** Be patient with yourself and accept your body's current state. Remember that somatic exercises are a journey of self-discovery and gradual improvement. Avoid pushing yourself too hard or expecting instant results.

Mindful awareness in somatic exercises promotes a deeper understanding of your body, its patterns, and its potential for change. It allows you to release tension, correct imbalances, and enhance your overall well-being. As you progress in your somatic practice, mindful awareness will become an integral part of your experience, enriching the benefits you derive from these exercises.

# CHAPTER 4

# Basic Somatic Exercises

## 4.1 Neck and Shoulder Release

The neck and shoulder region is a common area of tension and discomfort for many people, often due to factors like stress, poor posture, and excessive screen time. The Neck and Shoulder Release somatic exercise is designed to alleviate tension in this area and promote relaxation. Here's how to perform it:

**Preparation:**

1. Find a quiet, comfortable space to sit or stand. Ensure proper

lighting to observe your movements.

**Execution:**

1. Start by taking a few deep diaphragmatic breaths to relax your nervous system.

2. Begin with your head facing forward, and gently tilt your head to the right, bringing your right ear toward your right shoulder. Keep your movements slow and controlled.

3. As your right ear approaches your shoulder, notice any tension or discomfort in the left side of your neck and shoulder.

4. Inhale deeply as you gently tilt your head to the right. Feel the

stretch along the left side of
your neck and shoulder.

5. Exhale slowly and intentionally
relax the muscles on the left
side of your neck and shoulder.
Imagine the tension melting
away.

6. Inhale again, maintaining the
tilt to the right, but do not force
the stretch. Instead, focus on
the sensation of your breath and
the subtle release of tension
with each exhalation.

7. After several breaths, slowly
return your head to the neutral
position.

**Repeat the same process, tilting
your head to the left**:

1. Gently tilt your head to the left, bringing your left ear toward your left shoulder.

2. Observe any tension or discomfort in the right side of your neck and shoulder.

3. Inhale deeply while maintaining the tilt to the left, feeling the stretch along the right side.

4. Exhale slowly and intentionally relax the muscles on the right side of your neck and shoulder.

5. Inhale again, maintaining the tilt to the left, and focus on the sensation of your breath and the release of tension.

6. After several breaths, slowly return your head to the neutral position.

**Key Points:**

- Avoid any sudden or forceful movements; this exercise is about gentle release and awareness.

- Maintain a slow and deliberate pace to maximize the benefits of relaxation.

- Pay close attention to the sensations in your neck and shoulders as you perform the exercise, noticing how tension dissipates with each exhalation.

# 4.2 Spinal Wave

The Spinal Wave is a fundamental somatic exercise that helps release tension along the spine and improve overall spinal mobility. It's a flowing movement that encourages the natural undulating motion of the spine. Here's how to perform it:

**Preparation:**

1. Stand with your feet hip-width apart. Maintain a relaxed posture with your knees slightly bent and your arms hanging loosely by your sides.

**Execution:**

1. Begin by taking a few deep, diaphragmatic breaths to relax your body and center your focus.

2. As you inhale, slowly arch your spine backward, starting from the base of your spine (coccyx) and moving upward.

3. Allow your head to tilt slightly backward, but keep your chin

tucked to avoid straining your neck.

4. As you exhale, initiate a forward wave-like motion of your spine. Begin by tucking your chin to your chest and curving your upper back forward, followed by your mid-back and lower back.

5. Continue this wave-like motion down your spine, imagining each vertebra moving sequentially.

6. When you reach the end of your exhalation, let your body naturally round forward, relaxing into a gentle forward bend.

7. Inhale again and reverse the wave, starting from your coccyx and moving upward.

Slowly arch your spine backward, allowing your head to tilt back slightly.

**Repeat this spinal wave several times, synchronizing it with your breath**:

- Inhale: Arch backward, initiating from the base of your spine.

- Exhale: Initiate the forward wave-like motion, sequentially moving from the top of your spine to the bottom.

- Inhale: Arch backward again, reversing the wave.

**Key Points:**

- Maintain a slow and fluid motion throughout the exercise, allowing each vertebra to participate in the wave.

- Focus on the sensation of your spine moving and the release of tension with each wave.

- Perform this exercise with ease and without force, allowing your body to find its natural rhythm.

The Neck and Shoulder Release and the Spinal Wave are foundational somatic exercises that promote relaxation, release tension, and enhance body awareness. Incorporate these exercises into your somatic practice to experience increased mobility and a greater sense of well-being in your neck, shoulders, and spine.

## 4.3 Pelvic Tilt and Rotation

The Pelvic Tilt and Rotation exercise is designed to increase awareness of your pelvic region and improve its mobility. The pelvis plays a crucial role in overall posture and movement. This somatic exercise helps release tension and enhance the mobility of the pelvis. Here's how to perform it:

**Preparation:**

1. Find a comfortable, quiet space to stand with your feet hip-width apart. Maintain a relaxed posture with your knees slightly bent and your arms hanging loosely by your sides.

**Execution:**

1. Begin by taking a few deep, diaphragmatic breaths to relax

your body and center your focus.

2. Focus your attention on your pelvis. Imagine it as a bowl filled with water.

3. To initiate a pelvic tilt:

   - As you inhale, gently tilt your pelvis forward, as if you're pouring water out of the front of the bowl.

   - As you exhale, slowly return your pelvis to its neutral position.

4. Now, perform a pelvic rotation:

   - As you inhale, gently rotate your pelvis to the right, as if you're pouring water out of the right side of the bowl.

- As you exhale, return your pelvis to its neutral position.

- Repeat this rotation to the right several times while synchronizing it with your breath.

5. Perform the same pelvic rotation to the left:

  - As you inhale, gently rotate your pelvis to the left, as if you're pouring water out of the left side of the bowl.

  - As you exhale, return your pelvis to its neutral position.

  - Repeat this rotation to the left several times

while synchronizing it
with your breath.

**Key Points:**

- Maintain a slow, controlled
  pace throughout the exercise to
  maximize awareness and
  release of tension.

- Focus on the sensations in your
  pelvic region as you perform
  the pelvic tilt and rotation. Pay
  attention to how the movements
  affect your posture and
  alignment.

# 4.4 Arch and Flatten

The Arch and Flatten exercise is an
excellent way to address tension and
movement patterns in your spine,
particularly in the lumbar (lower
back) region. This somatic exercise

promotes flexibility and awareness of your spine's natural curvature. Here's how to perform it:

**Preparation:**

1. Find a comfortable, quiet space to lie on your back on a firm surface, such as a yoga mat or carpet. Bend your knees and place your feet flat on the floor, hip-width apart.

**Execution:**

1. Begin by taking a few deep, diaphragmatic breaths to relax your body and center your focus.

2. As you inhale, gently arch your lower back by lifting your pelvis off the floor. Imagine creating a small space between your lower back and the floor.

3. As you exhale, slowly return your pelvis to the floor, allowing your lower back to flatten against the surface.

4. Repeat this arch and flatten movement several times, synchronizing it with your breath:

   - Inhale: Arch your lower back, lifting your pelvis.

   - Exhale: Slowly return your pelvis to the floor, allowing your lower back to flatten.

**Key Points:**

- Keep your movements slow and deliberate, focusing on the sensation of your spine as it arches and flattens.

- Pay attention to the alignment of your pelvis and lower back during the exercise.

- Imagine each vertebra participating in the arch and flatten motion, creating space and mobility in your lower back.

The Pelvic Tilt and Rotation, along with the Arch and Flatten exercises, contribute to improved mobility and awareness in your pelvic and lumbar regions. Regular practice of these somatic exercises can help release tension, improve posture, and enhance your overall well-being by promoting a more balanced and supple spine.

# 4.5 Pandiculation: The Key to Somatic Exercises

Pandiculation is a fundamental concept and practice in somatic exercises. It serves as the key to unlocking the full benefits of somatic movement and is at the heart of somatic education. Pandiculation involves a deliberate and conscious contraction of a muscle or muscle group, followed by a slow and controlled release. This process is integral to resetting muscle length and function, ultimately leading to increased body awareness and relaxation. Here's how pandiculation works and how to incorporate it into your somatic practice:

**Understanding Pandiculation:**

- **Contraction:** To initiate pandiculation, you deliberately contract a specific muscle or group of muscles. This contraction is not forceful or intense but rather a gentle engagement to heighten your awareness of the targeted muscles.

- **Release:** After the contraction phase, you slowly and intentionally release the contracted muscles. The release phase is crucial as it allows the muscles to reset to their optimal resting length.

**Incorporating Pandiculation into Somatic Exercises:**

1. **Select a Targeted Muscle Group:** Choose a specific muscle or muscle group that you want to focus on during your somatic exercise. For

example, you might select the muscles of your neck and shoulders, your lower back, or your hips.

2. **Initiate the Contraction:** Begin by gently contracting the chosen muscle group. Focus on the sensation of the contraction and avoid any forceful or abrupt movements. The goal is to engage the muscles with awareness.

3. **Hold the Contraction:** Maintain the contraction for a few seconds, paying attention to the sensations in the engaged muscles. Notice any areas of tension or resistance.

4. **Slowly Release:** Begin to release the contraction slowly and deliberately. Imagine the

muscles lengthening and relaxing as you do so. This phase is where the magic of pandiculation occurs.

5. **Focus on Sensation:** Throughout the contraction and release, maintain mindful awareness of the sensations in the targeted muscle group. Be attentive to any changes in tension or discomfort.

6. **Repeat as Needed:** You can repeat the pandiculation process several times for the same muscle group or move on to another area of the body that requires attention. It's common to perform pandiculation during various somatic exercises, such as neck and shoulder releases or spinal waves.

**Benefits of Pandiculation:**

- **Improved Muscle Function:** Pandiculation helps reset muscle length and function, addressing issues related to chronic tension, tightness, or pain.

- **Enhanced Body Awareness:** By focusing on the sensations during pandiculation, you become more attuned to the specific muscle groups and their role in your movement patterns.

- **Promotes Relaxation:** The deliberate release of tension in pandiculation fosters relaxation, both physically and mentally, contributing to a more balanced and peaceful state of being.

- **Mind-Body Connection:** Pandiculation reinforces the mind-body connection by emphasizing conscious awareness of movement and muscle engagement.

Pandiculation is a central component of somatic exercises, and mastering this practice can significantly enhance the effectiveness of your somatic education. By incorporating pandiculation into your routine, you can release chronic tension, improve mobility, and develop a deeper understanding of your body, ultimately leading to greater overall well-being.

# CHAPTER 5

# Whole-Body Integration

## 5.1 Coordinating Movements

Whole-body integration in somatic exercises emphasizes the importance of coordinating movements and fostering a harmonious relationship between different muscle groups. The aim is to promote efficient and balanced movement patterns that allow the body to function optimally. Here's how to work on coordinating movements in your somatic practice:

**Mindful Sequencing:** Pay attention to the sequence of movements as you transition from one exercise or posture to another. Ensure that the transitions are smooth and deliberate, minimizing sudden or jerky movements.

**Sensory Feedback:** Use sensory feedback to guide your movements. Focus on the sensations in your body as you shift from one position to another, noticing any areas of tension, discomfort, or restriction. Sensory awareness helps you adjust your movements for optimal alignment and comfort.

**Breath and Movement:** Coordinate your breath with your movements. For example, inhale as you prepare for a movement, and exhale as you execute it. Breathing in harmony with your movements helps maintain a calm and centered state while improving coordination.

**Mind-Body Connection:** Continually reinforce the mind-body connection. Be present and fully engaged in each movement, ensuring that your body responds to your intentions and commands. This heightened awareness fosters better coordination.

**Progressive Sequencing:** Begin with simpler movements and gradually progress to more complex sequences as your somatic practice advances. Building coordination is a gradual process, and progressive sequencing helps avoid overwhelm.

# 5.2 Building Functional Patterns

Functional patterns in somatic exercises involve recreating natural, efficient movement patterns that are essential for everyday activities. The goal is to restore and reinforce these patterns to improve overall functionality. Here's how to work on building functional patterns:

**Functional Movement Exploration:** Explore everyday movements like bending, twisting, reaching, and walking mindfully. Pay attention to any areas of stiffness or discomfort and work on releasing tension and improving the ease of these movements.

**Functional Exercises:** Incorporate somatic exercises that mimic functional movements into your practice. For example, practice somatic squats to improve your ability to bend at the hips and knees with ease.

**Body Mechanics:** Focus on correct body mechanics during functional movements. Ensure that your posture is aligned, your core is engaged, and your movements are balanced and controlled. This helps prevent strain and injury during everyday activities.

**Mindful Daily Activities:** Extend somatic principles to your daily life. Be mindful of your posture, movement patterns, and muscle tension as you engage in routine tasks. Use somatic awareness to make adjustments for improved functionality.

Functional patterns are designed to enhance your ability to move and perform daily activities with greater ease and efficiency. By incorporating these patterns into your somatic practice, you can enjoy improved functionality and reduced risk of musculoskeletal issues.

## 5.3 Somatics for Posture Improvement

Posture improvement is a common goal in somatic exercises, as proper posture is essential for overall well-being and reduced risk of musculoskeletal problems. Here's how to focus on somatic for posture improvement:

**Postural Assessment:** Begin by assessing your current posture. Stand in front of a mirror and observe your alignment from the side, front, and back. Take note of any deviations from optimal posture, such as rounded shoulders, forward head position, or a tilted pelvis.

**Somatic Exercises for Posture:**
Incorporate somatic exercises that
target specific postural issues. For
example, if you have forward-rounded
shoulders, perform exercises that
release tension in the chest and
strengthen the upper back muscles.

**Pandiculation for Posture:** Use
pandiculation to reset the length and
function of muscles that contribute to
poor posture. Focus on contracting
and releasing specific muscle groups
involved in your postural deviations.

**Mindful Posture Correction:**
Throughout your day, maintain
mindful awareness of your posture.
Regularly check in with your body to
ensure that you're aligning yourself
optimally. Use somatic principles to
make micro-adjustments as needed.

**Somatic Education for Long-Term Posture:** Recognize that improving posture is an ongoing process. Somatic education provides you with the tools and awareness to continuously work on posture improvement throughout your life.

By integrating somatic exercises and awareness into your routine, you can make gradual improvements in your posture, reducing discomfort and promoting overall physical well-being. Whole-body integration in somatic practice extends beyond posture to encompass coordinated movements and functional patterns, enhancing your ability to move with ease and efficiency in everyday life.

# CHAPTER 6

# Somatic Exercises for Specific Issues

## 6.1 Stress and Tension Relief

Somatic exercises can be powerful tools for relieving stress and tension in the body. Here are some somatic exercises specifically designed to promote relaxation and reduce stress:

- **Full-Body Pandiculation:** Perform a full-body pandiculation to release tension throughout your body. Begin by contracting and releasing each major muscle group, starting from your toes and working your way up to your head. Focus on the sensation of tension melting away with each release.

- **Diaphragmatic Breathing:**
Practice diaphragmatic breathing to calm the nervous system. Lie on your back, place one hand on your chest and the other on your abdomen, and breathe deeply into your diaphragm. This exercise helps reduce the shallow chest breathing associated with stress.

- **Progressive Muscle Relaxation:** This exercise involves systematically tensing and then relaxing different muscle groups in the body. Start with your toes and work your way up to your head. As

66

you release tension in each muscle group, visualize stress and tension flowing out of your body.

- **Savasana (Corpse Pose):** In yoga, Savasana is a deeply relaxing pose that can be incorporated into somatic practice. Lie flat on your back, close your eyes, and focus on releasing tension from head to toe. Allow your body to feel heavy and supported by the ground.

## 6.2 Back Pain Relief

Somatic exercises can be highly effective in relieving back pain, whether it's in the upper, middle, or lower back. Here are some somatic exercises tailored to address various types of back pain:

- **Upper Back Tension Release:** Perform gentle neck and shoulder releases to address tension in the upper back. Focus on pandiculating the neck and shoulder muscles to release chronic tension.

- **Middle Back Mobility:** Use somatic spinal waves to improve mobility in the middle back. These flowing movements help release tension and promote a healthy range of motion in the thoracic spine.

- **Lower Back Pain Relief:** Practice arch and flatten exercises to alleviate lower back pain. This exercise helps reset the lumbar spine's natural curvature, releasing tension and improving alignment.

- **Full-Body Integration:** Incorporate full-body somatic exercises to address overall body tension that may contribute to back pain. A relaxed and coordinated body can alleviate stress on the back muscles.

# 6.3 Joint Mobility and Flexibility

Somatic exercises are valuable for improving joint mobility and flexibility. Here are some exercises to enhance the range of motion in specific joints:

- **Hip Mobility:** Perform somatic hip rotations to increase mobility in the hip joints. These movements help release tension and improve hip flexibility.

- **Shoulder Mobility:** Use gentle shoulder circles to promote mobility in the shoulder joints. Rotate your shoulders in small, controlled circles in both directions.

- **Spinal Flexibility:** Practice spinal waves to enhance the flexibility of the entire spine, from the cervical to the lumbar region. These flowing movements encourage a balanced and supple spine.

- **Knee Mobility:** Incorporate somatic knee bends to improve mobility in the knee joints. Gently bend and straighten your knees, paying attention to any areas of tension.

# 6.4 Improving Sleep with Somatics

Somatic exercises can also contribute to improved sleep by reducing stress and tension. Here are some exercises to help you relax and prepare for a restful night's sleep:

- **Savasana (Corpse Pose):** As mentioned earlier, Savasana is an excellent exercise for relaxation. Practice it before bedtime to release tension and calm your mind.

- **Progressive Muscle Relaxation:** Perform progressive muscle relaxation in bed as you wind down for sleep. Start with your toes and work your way up to your head, releasing tension and promoting relaxation.

- **Breathing Exercises:** Practice diaphragmatic breathing while lying in bed. Focus on slow, deep breaths to calm your nervous system and prepare your body for sleep.

- **Mindful Body Scan:** As you lie in bed, conduct a mindful body scan. Pay attention to each part of your body, releasing any tension or discomfort you may notice.

Somatic exercises for specific issues, such as stress relief, back pain, joint mobility, and sleep improvement, can be tailored to your individual needs. Incorporate these exercises into your daily routine to address specific concerns and enhance your overall well-being.

# CHAPTER 7

# Mindfulness and Somatics

## 7.1 Cultivating Mind-Body Awareness

Mind-body awareness is at the core of somatic practice. It involves developing a deep and conscious connection between your mind and body. Cultivating mind-body awareness is essential for understanding and transforming your movement patterns and overall well-being. Here's how to work on this aspect of somatic:

- **Mindful Attention:** Begin by paying mindful attention to your body's sensations, movements, and postures throughout the day. Notice how your body responds to different situations and activities.

- **Body Scanning:** Conduct regular body scans, where you systematically focus your attention on different parts of your body. This helps you identify areas of tension, discomfort, or imbalance.

- **Breath Awareness:** Use your breath as an anchor for mindfulness. Whenever you find your mind wandering, bring your focus back to your breath. Notice how your breath responds to changes in your body's state.

- **Interoception:** Develop interoception, which is the ability to perceive internal sensations. Notice your heartbeat, the feeling of your lungs expanding and contracting, and the subtle signals your body sends about its needs.

- **Non-Judgmental Observation:** Approach your body with non-judgmental observation. Instead of labeling sensations as "good" or "bad," simply observe and accept them as they are.

## 7.2 The Role of Mindfulness in Somatic Practice

Mindfulness is a foundational element of somatic practice. It serves several crucial roles in enhancing the effectiveness of somatics:

- **Awareness of Movement Patterns:** Mindfulness allows you to become acutely aware of your habitual movement patterns and postures. This awareness is essential for identifying and transforming inefficient or harmful habits.

- **Release of Tension:** Mindfulness enables you to identify areas of tension or discomfort in your body. By bringing conscious attention to these areas, you can release tension through pandiculation and other somatic techniques.

- **Improved Mind-Body Connection:** Mindfulness strengthens the mind-body connection. It helps you send clear and intentional signals to your muscles, promoting better control over your movements.

- **Stress Reduction:** Mindfulness promotes relaxation and reduces stress. By focusing your attention on the present moment, you can calm the nervous system and reduce the physical and mental effects of stress.

- **Enhanced Self-Awareness:** Through mindfulness, you gain a deeper understanding of your body, its limitations, and its potential for growth. This self-awareness empowers you to make informed choices about your somatic practice and overall health.

# 7.3 Mindful Movement

Mindful movement is a key aspect of somatic practice. It involves moving with deliberate awareness, paying attention to the sensations, alignment, and coordination of your body. Here's how to incorporate mindful movement into your somatic practice:

- **Slow and Controlled Movements:** Perform somatic exercises and movements slowly and with control. Avoid rushed or hasty motions. Instead, focus on each phase of the movement, paying attention to how your body responds.

- **Breath Awareness:** Coordinate your movements with your breath. Inhale as you prepare for a movement, and exhale as you execute it. This synchronization enhances your awareness of the mind-body connection.

- **Sensory Exploration:** Explore the sensations in your body as you move. Notice the way muscles engage and release, the texture of movement, and any areas of resistance or ease.

- **Focused Attention:** Direct your full attention to the movement at hand. Avoid distractions and multitasking. Engage your mind in the process, observing how each movement unfolds.

- **Intentional Alignment:** Pay careful attention to your alignment during movements. Ensure that your body is positioned optimally to minimize strain and promote efficient movement.

- **Mindful Everyday Activities:** Extend mindful movement to your daily life. Whether you're walking, sitting, or reaching for an object, practice awareness of your body's movements and postures in everyday activities.

Mindful movement enhances the benefits of somatic practice by deepening your connection to your body and promoting efficient, pain-free movement patterns. It's a valuable skill that can positively impact your physical and mental well-being both on and off the mat or exercise space.

# CHAPTER 8

# Advanced Somatic Practices

## 8.1 Exploring Further Somatic Exercises

Advanced somatic exercises offer a deeper exploration of mind-body connection, movement, and relaxation. These exercises often build upon the foundational practices covered earlier in the book. Here are some ways to explore further somatic exercises:

- **Progressive Complexity:** Gradually introduce more complex somatic movements into your practice. These exercises may involve greater coordination, integration of multiple muscle groups, or longer sequences.

- **Customization:** Tailor your somatic practice to address specific issues or goals. If you have particular areas of tension or stiffness, seek out somatic exercises designed to target those areas.

- **Guidance:** Consider seeking guidance from an experienced somatics instructor or practitioner. They can provide personalized instruction and feedback to enhance your practice.

## 8.2 Somatic Movement Sequences

Somatic movement sequences are choreographed series of somatic exercises designed to flow seamlessly from one movement to the next. These sequences offer a holistic approach to somatic practice and can be particularly beneficial for promoting relaxation, mobility, and overall well-being. Here's how to work with somatic movement sequences:

- **Select Sequences:** Explore different somatic movement sequences that align with your goals. Some sequences focus on specific issues like back pain relief, while others offer full-body integration and relaxation.

- **Flow and Breath:** Emphasize the connection between breath and movement as you flow through the sequence. Use your breath to guide the transitions between exercises and maintain a steady and mindful pace.

- **Mindful Attention:** Apply the principles of mindfulness to each movement within the sequence. Pay close attention to the sensations, alignment, and coordination of your body as you progress through the sequence.

- **Customization:** Modify or adapt sequences as needed to suit your individual needs and abilities. Over time, you can create your own somatic movement sequences based on your preferences and goals.

# CHAPTER 9

# Integrating Somatics into Daily Life

## 9.1 Incorporating Somatic Exercises into Your Routine

To maximize the benefits of somatic practice, it's essential to integrate it into your daily life. Here's how to incorporate somatic exercises seamlessly into your routine:

- **Morning Routine:** Start your day with a brief somatic exercise to awaken your body and mind. This can be a gentle movement sequence or a few minutes of breath and body awareness.

- **Desk Breaks:** If you have a sedentary job, take short somatic breaks throughout the day. Perform quick exercises or stretches to release tension and maintain mobility.

- **Pre-Sleep Practice:** Wind down in the evening with somatic exercises that promote relaxation and prepare your body for restful sleep.

- **Mealtime Mindfulness:** Practice mindful breathing or body scanning during meals to foster awareness of hunger and fullness cues, promoting healthier eating habits.

- **Incorporate Somatic Movement:** Include somatic

exercises in your workout routine or as part of your warm-up and cool-down to enhance overall movement quality.

## 9.2 Somatics for Stress Management

Somatics can be a powerful tool for managing stress. Here's how to use somatic principles for stress management:

- **Daily Relaxation:** Dedicate time each day to practice somatic exercises for relaxation. These may include full-body pandiculation, breath awareness, or gentle movement sequences.

- **Stress Check-Ins:** Regularly check in with your body to identify areas of tension or discomfort related to stress. Use somatic techniques to release this tension.

- **Mindful Response:** In moments of stress, pause and employ somatic principles to respond mindfully. Focus on your breath, release muscle tension, and ground yourself in the present moment.

- **Somatic Stress Reduction Techniques:** Explore specific somatic exercises designed to alleviate stress, such as neck and shoulder releases or deep breathing exercises.

# 9.3 Maintaining Long-Term Benefits

Somatic practice is most effective when it becomes a long-term commitment. Here's how to maintain the long-term benefits of somatic:

- **Consistency:** Stay consistent with your somatic practice. Incorporate it into your daily routine and view it as an ongoing journey of self-discovery and well-being.

- **Progressive Exploration:** Continually explore and deepen your somatic practice. Gradually introduce more advanced exercises and sequences to challenge and expand your abilities.

- **Mindful Living:** Extend the principles of somatic, such as mindful awareness and breath control, into all aspects of your life. Use these tools to navigate stress, enhance movement, and promote overall well-being.

- **Seek Guidance:** Consider seeking guidance from a certified somatic instructor or practitioner for periodic sessions to refine your practice and address specific concerns.

Integrating somatic practices into your daily life, you can experience sustained improvements in movement, relaxation, and overall health. It's a holistic approach that fosters a profound connection between your mind and body, leading to lasting well-being and vitality.

Made in the USA
Las Vegas, NV
04 December 2023

82123266R00056